Imposter Syndrome Busted
From Self-Doubt to Confidence

Author: Andrea Pluck

Cover design: Jeremy Pluck

First Published in 2025 in Australia by
Pluck Pluck Goose Publishing
1 Vaucluse Crescent
Bellevue Heights, South Australia 5050

ISBN: 978-0-9756253-9-2

Disclaimer

Andrea Pluck asserts her rights under the Copyright, Designs and Patents Act 1988 to be identified as the author of this book.

The content in this book/course is based on my personal experiences, professional knowledge, and research. It is intended for educational and informational purposes only and should not be considered medical, legal, or financial advice. While I strive to provide accurate and up-to-date information, I make no guarantees regarding the completeness, reliability, or applicability of the content to individual circumstances.

Massage therapy, business strategies, and professional development are highly individualised fields, and what works for one person may not work for another. Always consult with a qualified healthcare provider, legal professional, or business advisor before making decisions related to your health, practice, or career.

By engaging with this material, you acknowledge that I am not responsible for any outcomes—positive or negative—that may result from applying the concepts discussed. Your success depends on your unique situation, actions, and professional judgment.

Contents

Chapter 1: Understanding Imposter Syndrome 5

Chapter 2: The Impact of Imposter Syndrome 11

Chapter 3: Embracing your Strengths and Weaknesses 19

Chapter 4: Building Confidence 35

Chapter 5: Building a Professional Community 53

Chapter 6: Continuous Learning 65

Chapter 7: Ongoing Practice 77

Chapter 8: Continuing to Grow 85

Chapter 9: Your Personalised Action Plan 101

Additional Resources 111

Acknowledgments 117

About the Author 119

"You are so busy doubting yourself, while so many others are intimidated by your potential."

Author unknown

Chapter 1: Understanding Imposter Syndrome

"Just believe in yourself.

Even if you don't, pretend that you do, and at some point, you will."

Venus Williams

What is Imposter Syndrome

Imposter Syndrome was first identified in the 1970s by psychologists Dr. Pauline Clance and Dr. Suzanne Imes. They noticed that many high-achieving individuals—particularly women—often doubted their own abilities and felt like frauds, even when their success was evident to everyone else. Over time, research has shown that Imposter Syndrome affects people across all genders, professions, and walks of life.

At its core, Imposter Syndrome is characterised by feelings of self-doubt, fear of being exposed as a fraud, and a tendency to downplay achievements. It's not just a fleeting feeling—it's a pattern of thinking that can hold you back from reaching your full potential.

Understanding Imposter Syndrome is the first step toward overcoming it. By recognising these patterns in yourself, you can begin to challenge them. The goal isn't to eliminate self-doubt entirely—after all, it's natural to question yourself sometimes. Instead, it's about learning to manage those feelings, so they don't hold you back.

Common Signs and Symptoms

Imposter Syndrome can manifest in different ways, and not everyone experiences it in the same manner. However, some common signs include:

- Perfectionism: Setting impossibly high standards and feeling disappointed when you can't meet them.

- Overworking: Pushing yourself to exhaustion to prove your worth.

- Fear of Failure: Avoiding challenges or opportunities out of fear of not measuring up.

- Discounting Praise: Brushing off compliments or attributing success to luck.

Do any of these sound familiar? If so, don't worry—you're in good company.

As remedial therapists, these feelings may surface when working with clients, especially when we start questioning our own abilities.

I've personally struggled with perfectionism. Every project had to be flawless, every detail checked and re-checked, leaving me drained and, ironically, less productive. It wasn't until I recognised this pattern that I began to let go of unrealistic expectations and focus on meaningful progress instead of unattainable perfection.

This is what Imposter Syndrome used to look like for me:

- Chronic self-doubt

- Attributing success to external factors
- Fear of failure or being "found out"
- Downplaying accomplishments
- Overworking to prove worth

How do you experience Imposter Syndrome? Take a few minutes to reflect on your own experience of imposter syndrome (e.g. I tend to put off certain tasks, because I feel I am not confident enough to do them well (even though I've done all the training, and have three years of experience), and note them down on the following notes page.

Chapter 2: The Impact of Imposter Syndrome

> *"No one can make you feel inferior without your consent"*
>
> Eleanor Roosevelt

The Professional Impact

Imposter Syndrome doesn't just live quietly in the back of our minds—it seeps into every aspect of our lives. It affects how we approach our careers, our relationships, and even how we view ourselves

At work, Imposter Syndrome can appear in countless ways. Perhaps you hesitate to put yourself forward for promotions or exciting projects because you're convinced that you're not qualified. You might overwork yourself to "prove" your worth, fearing that any mistake will expose you as incompetent. On the other side, you might avoid challenges entirely, afraid of failing and confirming your internal doubts.

Professionally, imposter syndrome might prevent you from taking on new challenges, such as learning new techniques or expanding your practice. You might feel like you'll never be "good enough," leading to burnout from overwork or perfectionism.

The Personal Toll

Outside of work, Imposter Syndrome can damage your self-esteem and mental well-being. Constant self-doubt creates a cycle of anxiety, guilt, and emotional exhaustion, and second-guessing yourself. This mental load can impact your relationships and overall well-being. It can make it difficult to accept compliments, trust others' opinions of you, or feel deserving of love and respect. It's emotionally draining to constantly question yourself whether you are doing enough or truly deserve your accomplishments!

For many people, these feelings aren't fleeting—they're persistent. And over time, they can shape how you see yourself and your potential.

My Story

For me, the impact was subtle at first. I'd pass up chances to present at events or network with other professionals, thinking, "I'm not experienced enough," or "What could I possibly contribute?" Over time, though, I started realising how much I was limiting myself, and how those missed opportunities were holding me back from growing as a therapist.

It took me a long time to realise that Imposter Syndrome isn't a sign of weakness.

It helps to know that so many other people live with Imposter Syndrome. Some just don't know what it's called, but once you have that conversation, it's surprising how many others have it.

What about you?

Take a moment to think about your own experiences. Have you ever turned down an opportunity because you felt underqualified? Have you ever dismissed praise or felt like your achievements were just "luck"?

What are the triggers that amplify your self-doubt? What are those moments that make you question your abilities?

Jot down your thoughts in a journal or notebook, or on the next page. Identifying these patterns is the first step toward breaking free from them.

Once you understand how these feelings are impacting your daily life, you'll be one step closer to breaking free from their grip.

Self-awareness is key to overcoming imposter syndrome. When you can pinpoint what triggers these feelings of inadequacy, you can start to take control of them.

Chapter 3: Embracing your Strengths and Weaknesses

"Trust yourself. You know more than you think you do"

Johann Wolfgang von Goethe

Embracing your Weaknesses

Embracing your weaknesses can be one of the most empowering steps toward personal growth and success. It's easy to feel the pressure to present a perfect version of ourselves, but in reality, our weaknesses hold valuable lessons. Acknowledging them doesn't make us weak—it makes us human.

When we embrace our weaknesses, we give ourselves permission to be vulnerable, which is often when we learn the most. Weaknesses can be indicators of areas where we need growth or even points where we can ask for support from others. Instead of trying to hide them, we can use them as opportunities to build resilience and enhance our strengths.

Think of your weaknesses as a roadmap. Each one shows you a direction for improvement or self-reflection. Maybe you're not great at time management—

this could be a chance to explore new tools or strategies. Perhaps you struggle with saying no—learning how to set boundaries can turn this into a strength.

The key is to shift your perspective: what you once saw as a flaw can become a stepping stone to greater self-awareness and development. By embracing our weaknesses, we turn them into powerful catalysts for transformation.

Depression

I feel it's crucial to mention depression because the Imposter Syndrome and Depression can also be interconnected. The self-doubt, feelings of inadequacy, and fear of being "found out" that come with Imposter Syndrome can contribute to or exacerbate depression, making it important to acknowledge and address both. Recognising and seeking professional help for depression is an essential step in overcoming these challenges and fostering true self-acceptance. Depression is a condition that affects millions of people, yet it often goes unnoticed or misunderstood. It's not just feeling "down" or having a bad day—depression can take a profound toll on every aspect of life. The emotional heaviness, lack of motivation, and sense of isolation can make even the simplest tasks feel overwhelming.

One of the most crucial things to understand about depression is that it's not a sign of weakness or something you can simply "snap out of." It's a medical condition, and like any other illness, it deserves attention, care, and professional treatment.

Many people are hesitant to seek help due to stigma, fear, or not wanting to burden others. But the truth is, reaching out for support is one of the bravest things you can do. If you need to seek professional help, I have listed some resources towards the end of this book.

Remember, asking for help doesn't make you weak—it makes you strong. It's a commitment to your own well-being, and it's the beginning of a journey toward feeling better, one step at a time.

Embracing Your Strengths

By now, you've probably recognised some of the ways Imposter Syndrome has been showing up in your life. And if you're anything like me, you might be feeling a mix of relief ("I'm not alone!") and frustration ("Why can't I just shake this off?"). But what if I told you: you already have everything you need to start overcoming these feelings.

Learn to focus on something incredibly powerful—your strengths. Yes, you have them. And no, they're not flukes, luck, or happy accidents.

If there's one thing I've learned over the years, it's that every therapist has their own unique strengths—and that includes you. But when imposter syndrome kicks in, it can be hard to see those strengths clearly. You might start to feel like you don't bring anything special to the table or that you're somehow "less than" other therapists. I've felt this way too, especially when I was just starting out.

Believe me, you have skills, insights, and experiences that no one else has. Your combination of expertise, personality, and approach is what makes you stand out. You just need to learn to focus on identifying and embracing those strengths.

When you focus on your strengths, you're building a foundation of confidence. Instead of constantly worrying about what you lack, you start to see what you bring to the table. This shift in mindset allows you to show up more fully for your clients and feel more assured in your practice.

For me, it was realising that I had a knack for connecting with clients on a personal level. I might not have been the most experienced therapist in every technique, but I knew how to create a space where clients felt heard and supported. And that became my strength that made clients come back.

Why Embracing Strengths Feels So Hard

Let's face it: most of us seem to be experts at spotting our own weaknesses but terrible at recognising our strengths. Maybe you've been told not to "brag" or worry about coming across as arrogant. Or maybe your achievements just don't *feel* like achievements because they came naturally to you.

Your strengths and weaknesses can be your foundation for growth and confidence.

Discovering Your Strengths

So, how do you identify those strengths? Sometimes it's about paying attention to what lights you up, what others often compliment you on, or what comes effortlessly to you.

Do people frequently ask for your advice on a particular topic?

Are there tasks you find energising, even when they're challenging?

Have you ever been praised for something you dismissed as "no big deal"?

Take a moment to jot down your strengths. Even if it feels small, write it down. In fact, write down at least three.

Maybe you're excellent at hands-on techniques, providing personalised care that addresses your clients' specific needs. Or perhaps your strength lies in building strong client relationships and communication. You might also excel at adapting to new challenges or continuing to grow through ongoing education.

Everyone brings something unique to the table. By identifying your strengths, you can build confidence in your abilities and feel more secure in your role.

Seeking validation from others is natural—we all appreciate encouragement and recognition. However, when approval becomes the foundation of our self-worth, it can be a sign of deeper mental health struggles. Relying too heavily on external validation can lead to anxiety, low self-esteem, and even depression, as your sense of value becomes dependent on how others perceive you rather than on your own intrinsic worth.

This constant need for approval can be a destructive cycle, making you hesitant to take risks, voice your true opinions, or set boundaries for fear of disapproval. It can also leave you emotionally exhausted, as no amount of praise ever feels truly "enough" to fill the void of self-doubt.

Psychologist Dr. Ilene S. Cohen emphasises the pitfalls of seeking external validation:

"When we urgently aim to please other people, we're seeking approval of self from outside sources. And whenever we reach for something in the outside world to give us what we should be giving ourselves, we set ourselves up for disappointment." (Psychology Today, July 13, 2018).

True confidence comes from within—not from the approval of others but from knowing who you are, embracing your strengths, and accepting your imperfections. While feedback can be valuable, it should inform your growth, not define your worth. Breaking free from the need for constant validation allows you to live authentically, make decisions based on your own values, and build resilience in the face of criticism or rejection.

Owning Your Strengths and Weaknesses

Owning your strengths and weaknesses is about embracing who you are—both the parts you're proud of and the areas where you have room to grow. When you acknowledge your strengths, you give yourself permission to shine and use them to your advantage. These are the qualities that set you apart, the skills you bring to the table, and the achievements you've earned through hard work.

Owning your weaknesses is equally important. It's about being honest with yourself and recognising that perfection isn't the goal—growth is. By facing your weaknesses without shame, you can take proactive steps to improve, whether that's learning new skills, seeking help, or simply accepting that it's okay to not have all the answers.

Identifying strengths and weaknesses is one thing, but owning them? That's where the real work begins. Owning your strengths and weaknesses means allowing yourself to acknowledge your talents without qualification. It means silencing that inner critic that says, *"Anyone could have done this."*

Together, owning both your strengths and weaknesses creates a balanced, authentic version of yourself. It frees you from the pressure to be perfect and allows you to be more confident, self-aware, and ready to take on whatever comes your way.

Remember those strengths you wrote down in the last chapter? Now, for each one, write a short sentence about how you've demonstrated it recently.

Here are some of my own to help you get started:

Strength: Organisation

Example: I created ways for one of my mentees to be more organised and achieve her goals more efficiently.

Strength: Creativity

Example: I came up with an innovative solution during a challenging meeting.

Small moments count. Celebrate them.

Once you've identified your strengths and weaknesses, it's important to actively remind yourself of them, especially when imposter syndrome starts creeping in. Identifying strengths as well as weaknesses and working through accepting both are very important aspects of who you are. Failure is essential for growth. Just because you failed at something, doesn't mean it's a weakness. It means you need to focus some energy on improving in that area, so you fail less. Self-affirmation exercises can be incredibly helpful here. You could try to keep a "strengths journal." Each week, take a few minutes to write down moments where you felt confident or where you used one of your strengths. It's a simple practice, but over time, it builds up your sense of self-worth.

Or you could create a strengths mantra. This is a short, empowering statement that you can repeat to yourself when self-doubt arises. For example, "I am skilled at connecting with my clients and providing them with personalised care." These small but powerful reminders can help you shift your mindset and embrace the value you bring as a therapist.

What works for me? Whenever I'm driving in the car to a new workshop or presentation, I like to play the song "The only way is up" by Yazz at full volume. It's inspirational and helps me shift my mindset.

Embracing your strengths doesn't mean you have to ignore areas where you can grow, but it's about building on the solid foundation you already have. It's about recognising that you bring something valuable to the table—something that no one else can replicate. So, take some time to reflect on your unique strengths and think about how you can lean into them more fully in your practice.

You're already more capable than you think. Your strengths are there—you just need to claim them.

Chapter 4: Building Confidence

"If we all did the things we are capable of doing, we would literally astound ourselves."

Thomas Edison

Building Confidence Through Action

Overcoming Imposter Syndrome isn't about silencing every doubt forever—it's about developing tools and strategies to manage those thoughts when they inevitably pop up. Confidence isn't something you either *have* or *don't have*—it's something you need to *build (and maintain)*, one step, one small win, one brave moment at a time.

You can start building that confidence foundation with practical steps, meaningful connections, and a mindset that works *with* you instead of against you.

Small Wins, Big Impact

Something I've learned over time: confidence doesn't come from one big, grand achievement. It comes from stacking up all those small wins—

consistently. You know, those little moments when you step out of your comfort zone, finish something you've been avoiding, or speak up even when your voice shakes.

Each of those moments is proof. Proof that you're capable, that you *can* do hard things, and that you deserve a seat at the table.

In this section, I want to show you how to identify and celebrate those small wins, build habits that set you up for success, and shift your focus from what went wrong to what went *right*.

The Power of the Mind

Ah, mindset. It's one of those buzzwords we hear all the time, but when it comes to Imposter Syndrome, it's *everything*.

Your thoughts shape your reality—and I don't mean that in a "just think positive" kind of way. I mean recognising when your inner voice is feeding you lies (*"You're not good enough"* or *"You just got lucky"* or *"They're just being polite"*) and challenging those thoughts head-on.

If Imposter Syndrome thrives on anything, it's a mindset of self-doubt and fear. The way we talk to ourselves, the stories we tell about our abilities, and the expectations we place on ourselves all shape how we perceive our value. To overcome Imposter Syndrome, we need to shift our mindset.

Sadly though, mindset shifts don't happen overnight. They're built slowly, through consistent effort and self-awareness.

Mindset is like a lens through which you view the world—and yourself. When Imposter Syndrome takes hold, this lens becomes clouded, magnifying your flaws and downplaying your strengths. A shift in mindset allows you to see a clearer, more balanced picture of who you are and what you bring to the table.

Psychologist Carol Dweck's research into fixed and growth mindsets provides a useful framework for understanding this. A fixed mindset assumes that your abilities are set in stone, that you're either "good enough" or you're not. In contrast, a growth mindset sees challenges as opportunities to develop and improve.

When Imposter Syndrome convinces you that you're not ready or not capable, it's often rooted in a fixed mindset. Adopting a growth mindset means recognising that your skills are not static; they can grow with effort, learning, and perseverance. It's a perspective that shifts your focus from fear of failure to excitement for growth.

Reframing Negative Thoughts

Negative thoughts are often automatic and critical. Instead of accepting them as facts, you can learn to challenge them. A significant part of shifting your mindset involves recognising and changing the way you respond to negative thoughts.

For example, if you catch yourself thinking, *"I'm not qualified to be here,"* pause and ask yourself why you feel that way. Then reframe the thought by focusing on evidence of your competence, such as the effort you put in or the unique skills you bring. You might say to yourself, *"I've worked hard for this opportunity, and my perspective adds value here."*

This practice doesn't mean ignoring all doubts or forcing yourself into blind positivity. It's about finding a balanced perspective—one that acknowledges challenges without letting them overshadow your accomplishments.

Instead of seeing failure as proof of inadequacy, see it as a lesson. Ask yourself, *"What can I learn from this?"*

Ask better questions. Instead of asking, *"Why am I so bad at this?"* ask, *"What can I do to get better?"*

Celebrate progress, not perfection. Every small step counts. Did you try something new? Did you learn something you didn't know yesterday? Celebrate that.

Shifting your mindset isn't an overnight thing—it takes practice. But every time you choose curiosity over self-criticism, you're moving in the right direction.

Cultivating Self-Compassion

We often hold ourselves to impossible standards, expecting perfection while extending grace to others. Yes, I admit I am guilty of this. Shifting your mindset requires developing self-compassion, treating yourself with the same kindness you would offer a friend.

When you catch yourself being overly critical, pause and reflect. Would you speak to a loved one in the same way? If not, take a moment to reframe the criticism into something more constructive. For instance, instead of saying, *"I'm terrible at this,"* you might say, *"This is a skill I'm still learning, and that's okay."*

Self-compassion is a skill that grows with practice. Over time, it can soften the harsh voice of self-doubt and create space for growth and acceptance.

Practicing Gratitude

When we think of gratitude, we often think of and acknowledge what's good around us. But it's also about recognising what's good within you.

One way to do this is by writing down three things you're proud of or grateful for about yourself each day. They don't have to be monumental—small wins count, too.

At the end of the day, I like to take a moment to reflect on things I feel proud of or grateful for—especially when those self-doubts creep in. For example, there was a day last week when I finished writing a particularly challenging section of another book. It wasn't perfect, but I put in the effort, and that mattered.

Another moment came when a former student reached out to thank me for something I taught her years ago. It reminded me that the work I do has a ripple effect—it helps people in ways I might not always see.

Finally, I'm grateful for the courage I've built to tackle Imposter Syndrome head-on. It's not always easy, but taking this step to share my journey with you is something I genuinely value.

Visualising Success

Visualisation is a powerful tool for mindset shifts. When you picture yourself succeeding—not through luck, but because of your hard work and skill—you train your brain to see success as attainable. Do you remember that movie "Cool Runnings" about the Jamaican bobsled team? They would close their eyes and imaging themselves flying down the track, feeling the speed and the turns. This helped them to stay calm and focused during the race. Whenever I think of visualisation it reminds me of this.

Take a few moments each day to imagine yourself achieving a specific goal. See yourself navigating challenges with confidence and feeling that you have achieved something meaningful. It's like a mental rehearsal. The more vividly you visualise success, the more your brain begins to believe in the possibility.

Surrounding Yourself with Positivity

The people you surround yourself with play a significant role in shaping your mindset. If you're constantly around individuals who doubt or diminish you, it's easy to internalise those messages. Instead, seek out colleagues, and friends who uplift and inspire you. It's important to have positive people around you, but it is also important to have people around you who will communicate truth to you. Friends who will offer constructive criticism, as well as positive encouragement. Balance is important for staying true to yourself, and for keeping both feet firmly on the ground.

A truly supportive peer network is much like an anchor and a buoy. A network to which you can tether, where you can remain yourself (floating and bobbing around where you will), but where you are firmly attached to the sea floor so you won't drift off in dangerous currents and swells. They are also there for when you need help to keep your head above the water. Their encouragement helps you build confidence and challenges the narrative of self-doubt.

Moving Forward

Shifting your mindset isn't about banishing every doubt forever—it's about learning to manage and reframe those doubts when they arise. With self-awareness, compassion, and a focus on growth, you can begin to change the way you see yourself and your potential.

This work is ongoing, but every small step you take builds momentum. Mindset shifts are about progress, not perfection.

> Overcoming Imposter Syndrome isn't about being fearless—it's about being brave *despite* your fears.

Embracing a Growth Mindset

You've probably heard the term *growth mindset* thrown around a lot, but let's keep it simple. A growth mindset is the belief that your abilities, intelligence, and skills aren't fixed—they can grow and improve with time, effort, and practice.

This mindset isn't about being endlessly positive or pretending everything is fine. It's about changing the *story* you tell yourself when you hit a roadblock.

Understanding How We Learn and Adapt

Embracing a growth mindset means recognising that intelligence isn't fixed—it evolves with effort, experience, and learning. A key concept in understanding this is the distinction between **crystallised intelligence** and **fluid intelligence**, two types of cognitive abilities that shape how we process information and solve problems.

Crystallised intelligence is the accumulation of knowledge, facts, and experiences we gain over time. It's what allows us to recall information, use vocabulary effectively, and apply learned skills. Think of it as the wisdom that grows as we age—it's built through education, reading, and lived experiences.

Fluid intelligence, on the other hand, is our ability to think flexibly, solve new problems, and adapt to unfamiliar situations without relying on prior knowledge. It's what helps us think critically, see patterns, and tackle challenges creatively. Unlike crystallised intelligence, which strengthens over time, fluid intelligence tends to peak in early adulthood and may decline with age—though it can be maintained and even improved with practice.

Both forms of intelligence are essential, and a **growth mindset** encourages us to cultivate both. While crystallised intelligence provides a strong foundation of knowledge, fluid intelligence allows us to innovate and adapt. By continually challenging ourselves—learning new skills, engaging in problem-solving, and staying curious—we can enhance both types of intelligence and keep growing at any stage of life.

Chapter 5: Building a Professional Community

"Alone, we can do so little; together, we can do so much"

Helen Keller

Building a Professional Community

As therapists, we often work one-on-one with clients, which can make our professional lives feel solitary at times. But when you build connections with other therapists, you create a support system where you can share challenges, celebrate successes, and learn from one another.

For me, having a community of like-minded therapists has been invaluable. When I've felt uncertain or overwhelmed, I've had peers who were there to offer advice, encouragement, and even just a listening ear. It's a reminder that we're all in this together.

One of the most powerful ways to overcome Imposter Syndrome is to realise you're not alone—and the best way to do that is by surrounding yourself with genuine individuals who are willing to help.

When you're part of a professional community, you have access to shared experiences and stories that remind you *you're not the only one*. You are able to get practical advice from people who've been where you are.

A support system celebrates your wins and lifts you up during your struggles.

One of the most effective ways to build a community is to create or join a support group. This could be a formal peer supervision group where you meet regularly to discuss cases and provide feedback, or it could be an informal group where you share ideas and encourage each other.

When I first started my practice, I joined a peer group of local therapists. We'd meet monthly, and those meetings quickly became a lifeline for me. We'd talk through tough cases, celebrate small victories, and most importantly, remind each other that we weren't alone in our challenges.

Whether it's emotional support, shared learning, or simply having someone to talk to, your community can help you navigate the ups and downs of your career.

Take some time to think about how you can expand or deepen your professional network. Reach out to colleagues, join online groups, or attend an industry event. The more connected you feel to others in your field, the less alone you'll feel in your struggles.

In the next chapter we'll look at practical strategies for overcoming imposter syndrome, including cognitive behavioral techniques and mindfulness practices. But for now, focus on building your support network—you might be surprised at how much it helps.

Networking with Professionals

Networking with like-minded professionals is one of the most powerful ways to grow your career, gain new insights, and feel supported in your field. Whether you're looking for advice, collaboration opportunities, or just a sense of belonging, building connections with others who share your passion can open doors to endless possibilities.

"You have no friends. You have no enemies. You only have teachers" - Buddhist Proverb

I think it's important when talking about relationships. It helps to re-frame interactions with individuals and groups, particularly those people whose attributes you aspire to. In approaching an interaction from the perspective of learning; you quite often can pay more attention to information and cues during the interaction, than on how you appear to them. It can also help with addressing issues you may have with others, by maintaining a calm and objective mindset.

It's about staying curious.

In Australia, there are numerous resources to help you connect with others in your industry. Professional associations like Massage & Myotherapy Australia and the Association of Massage Therapists offer memberships that include networking events, workshops, and access to forums where you can share knowledge and experiences. Attending conferences, or state-based wellness or health expos, is another excellent way to meet like-minded professionals in a collaborative and educational environment.

Online platforms also provide opportunities to connect, especially in a geographically diverse country like Australia. Joining online groups or participating in forums tailored to your profession can help you engage with peers, even if you're in a remote location.

Social media groups, such as online communities for massage therapists or allied health professionals, often provide a space to ask questions, share experiences, and support each other.

Networking is about building mutually beneficial relationships. When you show genuine interest in others' work and are willing to share your own experiences and knowledge, you'll find that your professional network becomes an invaluable source of growth and inspiration.

Networking doesn't have to feel stiff or transactional. In fact, the best networking happens naturally—through shared interests, conversations, and mutual respect. Here are some tips:

Networking can be done by attending workshops, conferences, or online events related to your field.

Don't be afraid to introduce yourself—most people are just as nervous about networking as you are.

Follow up with connections. A quick "It was great meeting you!" email or message can go a long way.

Creating Safe Spaces for Support

Creating safe spaces for support is necessary in fostering meaningful connections and nurturing professional growth. A safe space is more than just a physical environment—it's a mindset and culture where individuals feel comfortable sharing their experiences, seeking advice, and expressing vulnerabilities without fear of judgment or criticism.

For professionals, especially in fields like massage therapy or health and wellness, these spaces provide an opportunity to discuss challenges, celebrate achievements, and build resilience. Safe spaces encourage open conversations about issues like imposter syndrome, burnout, or professional dilemmas, helping individuals feel heard and validated.

Creating such spaces starts with establishing trust. When networking or collaborating, lead with empathy and respect. Listen actively, avoid making assumptions, and offer support in a way that aligns with the needs of others. For example, peer support groups or accountability circles can be valuable tools. These groups, often facilitated in person or online, create structured opportunities to share and reflect, ensuring everyone has a voice.

In Australia, we have initiatives like mentorship programs within professional associations, informal meet-ups through social media groups, or regional practitioner networks are great ways to cultivate these supportive environments. You can also initiate your own safe spaces by organising small, regular gatherings with peers where the focus is on mutual growth and encouragement.

By contributing to or creating these spaces, you're building a network and fostering a culture of support that benefits the entire professional community.

Safe spaces aren't just about physical environments—they're about creating a culture where honesty, vulnerability, and encouragement are the norm.

This could mean:

- Finding (or creating!) a peer support group.

- Joining online forums or communities where people openly discuss professional challenges.

- Simply reaching out to a trusted colleague when you need advice or support.

When you surround yourself with people who *get it*, you'll find that those nagging self-doubts start to lose their power.

Moving Forward

Confidence doesn't mean you'll never feel fear or self-doubt again. It means you'll know how to keep moving forward *despite* those feelings.

And most importantly, building confidence isn't about being perfect—it's about showing up, trying again, and recognising your own progress.

Keep going. You've got this.

Chapter 6: The Importance of Continuous Learning

"Rise up and greet your higher self."

Kendall Toole

The Importance of Continuous Learning

You know that saying, *"The more I learn, the more I realise how much I don't know"*? Yes, I feel that. And honestly, I think there's something really beautiful about it. Continuous learning isn't about stockpiling facts or trying to prove you're the smartest person in the room. It's about staying curious, staying open, and reminding yourself that growth is a continuous path.

One of the sneakiest tricks Imposter Syndrome plays on us is convincing us that we should already *know everything*. That if we don't have all the answers right now, then we're somehow failing. But no one knows *everything*. Not the most experienced professionals in your industry, not those polished experts you admire online. And honestly? That's a *good* thing. It means there's always room to grow, evolve, and discover new things about yourself and your practice.

Continuous learning can be empowering. There are opportunities for learning everywhere.

Professional development builds confidence

Here's something I've noticed: growth doesn't happen when we're stuck in our comfort zones. Sure, staying in familiar territory feels safe—but it's also where Imposter Syndrome loves to linger. Real growth happens when we stretch ourselves, when we admit we don't know something and decide to learn anyway.

Continuous learning isn't just about professional growth (though that's a big part of it).

First, it increases your competence—you'll feel more equipped to handle a wider range of client needs. Learning new techniques and approaches also helps you build trust with your clients, showing them that you're committed to providing the best possible care.

Investing in your ongoing education can also contribute to your career's longevity. By staying current with industry standards, you'll continue to grow professionally, ensuring you remain competitive and relevant.

It's also about personal growth—feeling more confident in your abilities, embracing your curiosity, and realising that not knowing something doesn't mean you're not good enough. It just means you haven't learned it *yet*.

Continuous learning keeps your skills sharp and relevant in a constantly changing world. It builds confidence because knowledge is *empowering*. It normalises not knowing everything and replaces fear with curiosity. And it helps you adapt when life throws unexpected challenges your way.

But maybe the most important thing? Learning helps you embrace the idea that you're *allowed* to be a work in progress. You're not supposed to have it all figured out—and that's okay.

Finding Opportunities to Learn

Opportunities to learn are *everywhere*. Seriously, once you start looking, you'll notice them popping up all over the place. And no, it doesn't always mean signing up for expensive courses or heading back to school. Attending conferences or industry events provide great learning opportunities, as do books, research papers and industry journals. Or you may like to take an online course – there are so many affordable options out there. Podcasts are great for when you're commuting or on the go (or in my case, when folding the laundry).

Even having a coffee with someone you admire can provide you with a great learning opportunity.

Some of the best learning happens when you just *start*. Volunteer for a project that pushes you outside your comfort zone. Try a new approach at work. Take on a challenge that makes you a little nervous.

The point isn't to collect certifications or rack up "proof" of your expertise. It's about staying curious and letting yourself grow—one step at a time.

Balancing Learning with Self-Compassion

Okay, quick reality check: you don't have to learn *everything* right now. It's so easy to fall into the trap of thinking you need to master every skill, read every book, and say yes to every opportunity. Learning is a lifelong practice, not a race.

Give yourself permission to learn at your own pace, take breaks when you need them, and celebrate what you *have* learned, instead of obsessing over what you *haven't*.

Some seasons of life are for deep learning, and others are for resting and applying what you've already learned. Both are valuable. Allow time to apply what you've learned.

A Learning Plan That Works for You

You don't need a perfectly mapped-out five-year learning plan (unless that's your thing—then go for it!). But having a loose idea of where you want to grow can be helpful.

It helps to ask yourself what areas you want to improve in, personally or professionally. Think about what sparks your curiosity or excites you. Write down one small step you can take this month to learn something new

Maybe it's reading one book, attending one webinar, or setting aside an hour a week for professional development. Keep it simple, keep it doable, and most importantly—keep it fun.

Personally, I like to revisit this every so often.

Moving Forward

Here's what I want you to remember: continuous learning isn't about proving your worth. It's about embracing growth, staying curious, and reminding yourself that it's *okay* not to know everything. You're not supposed to.

I hope you feeling a little more inspired to adopt a growth mindset and equipped with ideas for finding learning opportunities.

Most of all, I hope you feel confident in creating a learning rhythm that fits *your* life.

Pick a book, listen to a podcast, or sign up for an online course that excites you. Remember, every small step adds up over time.

Chapter 7: Ongoing Practice

"Doubt kills more dreams than failure ever will."

Suzy Kassem

Setting Realistic Goals

Goal setting can feel like one of those things we *know* we should do, but often avoid because it feels overwhelming or even pointless. Maybe you've set goals before, only to lose momentum halfway through. Clear, actionable goals aren't just wishful thinking—they're powerful tools for progress.

Why SMART Goals Work

You've probably heard of SMART goals before: Specific, Measurable, Achievable, Relevant, and Time-Bound. It's a framework that transforms your goals into clear actionable steps. But let's break it down together in a way that feels practical and, dare I say, doable.

Specific: Instead of saying, *"I want to improve my skills,"* try something like, *"I *want to complete an advanced course on lymphatic drainage techniques."*

Measurable: How will you know when you've achieved your goal? Will you have a certificate, a set number of completed case studies, or client feedback?

Achievable: Set goals that stretch you but don't set you up for burnout. For example, *"I'll dedicate one hour every Friday to professional development."*

Relevant: Make sure your goals align with what truly matters to you. If growing your practice is a priority, focus on goals that directly support that.

Time-Bound: Deadlines are your friend! Instead of "someday," aim for *"I'll complete this course within three months."*

When you use this approach, your goals stop being abstract ideas and start becoming actionable steps.

Big Goals, Small Steps

Even the most well-defined goal can feel intimidating if it seems too big. Break it down into smaller, more manageable pieces.

For example:

Big Goal: Complete an advanced certification course.

Smaller Steps:

Research course options.

Choose and enroll in the right program.

Set aside weekly study time.

Complete one module per week.

Celebrate each milestone!

Each small win fuels your momentum and gives you a sense of accomplishment.

Staying Accountable

We've all experienced the initial burst of enthusiasm when setting a goal, only to see it fade away after a few weeks. So, how do you stay on track?

Write It Down: Physically writing your goals down makes them more real and harder to ignore. Keep them somewhere visible—a sticky note on your desk, a journal, or even a vision board.

Check In Regularly: Schedule regular check-ins with yourself. Weekly or monthly reviews can help you assess your progress and make adjustments.

Find an Accountability Partner: Share your goals with a trusted friend, or colleague. When someone else knows what you're working toward, you're more likely to follow through.

Celebrate Progress: Don't wait until the finish line to celebrate. Acknowledge the little victories along the way—they're just as important.

Flexibility is Key

Here's the truth: life happens. Unexpected challenges pop up, priorities shift, and some goals might need adjusting. And that's okay! Flexibility doesn't mean giving up—it means adapting.

If something isn't working, don't be afraid to revisit your goal, tweak your timeline, or adjust your approach. The key is to stay committed to the *why* behind your goal, even if the *how* changes.

Your Roadmap to Success

Setting goals isn't about adding more pressure to your plate—it's about giving yourself a roadmap to success. It's about knowing where you're headed and having the confidence to take one step at a time.

So, let me ask you: *What's one goal you've been putting off because it feels too big or too vague?*

Take a moment, write it down, and start breaking it into smaller steps. You'll be amazed at what you can achieve when you give yourself clarity, structure, and a little grace along the way.

Keep moving forward—you've got this!

Chapter 8: Continuing to Grow

"Don't trade your authenticity for approval."

Anonymous

Finding Opportunities to Learn

Learning isn't always about sitting in a classroom or completing a course—it's about staying curious, asking questions, and seeing every experience as a chance to grow. And here's the thing: opportunities to learn are everywhere, but sometimes we miss them because we're so focused on "big" milestones like certifications or degrees.

Every day is an opportunity to learn.

Learning in Everyday Moments

One of the most valuable lessons I've learned is that growth often happens in the small, seemingly insignificant moments. Maybe it's a client who asks a question you don't immediately know the answer to. Instead of brushing it off, take a moment to research, ask a colleague, or dive into a resource. That single question could lead you down a path of discovery that strengthens your expertise.

Stay Curious in Conversations

Every conversation is a chance to learn something new—whether it's with a peer, a mentor, or even a client. When someone shares their approach to a challenge or their perspective on a problem, listen deeply. Ask follow-up questions. People love to share their knowledge, and you'll often walk away with an insight you didn't expect.

Look for Gaps in Your Knowledge

Sometimes, growth starts with admitting where you feel less confident. Instead of avoiding those areas, lean into them. Is there a technique in your practice you wish you were better at? A business skill you've been meaning to develop? A topic your clients keep bringing up that you don't know much about? Those "gaps" are golden opportunities—they're basically signposts pointing you toward your next growth area.

One of the most empowering things you can do for your growth is to get curious about what you don't know. I know, it sounds counterintuitive—most of us focus on what we *do* know to feel confident. But identifying gaps in your knowledge isn't about highlighting weaknesses; it's about opening doors to new possibilities.

For instance, think about an area in your work or personal life where you often feel stuck or unsure. Maybe it's a technical skill, like mastering a new software program, or something more specific, like improving your communication with clients or colleagues. These "gaps" aren't limitations—they're opportunities waiting to be explored.

When I first started exploring Imposter Syndrome, I realised I didn't fully understand its psychological roots. Instead of letting that intimidate me, I leaned into learning. I read books, attended workshops, and spoke with experts. That process didn't just fill the gap; it gave me the confidence to turn what I learned into something meaningful—this very resource you're reading now.

Start by asking yourself "What skills or knowledge could help me feel more capable or confident in a specific area?" Then take small steps to address them.

Remember, it's not about knowing everything—it's about knowing where to grow. And that shift in perspective can be incredibly liberating.

Embrace Challenges

Let's talk about challenges—not as obstacles to be feared, but as opportunities to grow. I get it: facing challenges can feel overwhelming, especially when Imposter

Syndrome is whispering in your ear that you're not ready or capable.

It's easy to stick with what feels comfortable. But real learning happens when you step slightly outside your comfort zone. Say yes to that speaking opportunity, even if it feels scary. Take on a challenging client case, even if it stretches your skills. Every time you push past that initial hesitation, you grow—and you're expanding your skills, your resilience, and your confidence.

I remember a time when I was asked to step in to lead a workshop for a group of professionals far more experienced than I was. My initial reaction? Panic. I almost said no, convinced that someone else would do a better job. But instead, I decided to approach it as a learning experience. I prepared thoroughly, leaned into my strengths, and reminded myself that even if I stumbled, I'd still come out of it with new insights. And you know what? That challenge ended up being a turning point for me.

Embracing challenges doesn't mean you won't feel nervous or uncertain—it means you move forward anyway, trusting that you'll learn and grow along the way. The more you do this, the more evidence you'll have to counter those nagging doubts. Challenges aren't there to prove your worth; they're there to help you discover it.

So the next time you're faced with a daunting task or opportunity, pause and reframe it. Instead of asking, *"What if I fail?"* try asking, *"What might I learn?"* It's not about being perfect—it's about being brave enough to try.

Be Open to Different Learning Styles

You're heard of "one size fits all". Well, learning isn't like that, and being open to different styles can make all the difference.

Maybe you've always thought of yourself as a visual learner, or someone who prefers hands-on experiences. That's great! But what if there are other approaches you haven't explored yet that could enhance your understanding or open new doors?

I used to believe that traditional workshops and lectures were the only way I absorbed knowledge effectively. I would usually sit in the back row because that's where I would feel comfortable. Then, I read somewhere that you learn most when you are slightly uncomfortable. Actually, I'm not sure if that's the case for everyone, but it worked for me. From then on I usually find a seat where I feel slightly uncomfortable. I still do this to this very day.

I also found out that I could learn quite a lot from discussion groups.

Turns out the key is to experiment!

Try reading books or articles, watching videos, joining discussion groups, or even shadowing a colleague. If something doesn't click, that's okay—it's about finding what works for you. By embracing different learning styles, you're discovering how to engage with it in ways that resonate most with you.

Sometimes, stepping out of your comfort zone in how you learn can feel just as rewarding as the knowledge itself. And the best part? You're building a toolkit of diverse methods that will support you throughout your personal and professional growth.

Not everyone learns the same way, and that's okay! Some people love structured courses, while others prefer diving into books, attending workshops, or even just having deep conversations with peers. The important thing is to stay open to different methods. You might discover that you love hands-on workshops or that podcasts fit perfectly into your morning routine.

Create Your Own Opportunities

Sometimes, waiting for the "perfect" opportunity means waiting forever. I've learned that some of the most rewarding experiences in my life didn't just fall into my lap—I had to create them. It can feel daunting at first, but taking initiative often opens doors you didn't even know existed.

Creating your own opportunities starts with identifying what excites you or aligns with your goals. Maybe there's a gap in your industry that you're uniquely equipped to fill. Or perhaps you've noticed a lack of networking events in your area and decide to start one yourself. I remember wanting to deepen my skills in a specific area of practice, but there wasn't a course that fit my needs. Instead of giving up, I reached out to a circle of support and designed a self-study plan with their guidance.

The beauty of creating opportunities is that it puts you in the driver's seat. It could be as simple as volunteering for a project at work, offering to mentor a colleague, or collaborating on a community initiative. The effort you invest builds your skills and shows others your drive and creativity.

Don't wait for someone else to create the perfect chance for you. Look at your goals, think creatively, and ask yourself, "What can I start today to move closer to where I want to be?" You might be surprised at the doors you open when you take that first step.

Sometimes, the learning opportunities you need don't exist yet—and that's your cue to create them. Start a peer study group, host a discussion night with colleagues, or propose a training session in your workplace. When you take ownership of your learning journey, you'll often find others who are eager to join you.

Revisit your motivation

Every now and then, it's important to revisit our initial motivation for becoming a therapist. For some, it was a natural transition from a previous career. For others, a complete shift in personal and professional goals. Each therapist has their own unique journey, shaped by their aspirations and values.

Financial success is often seen as a primary measure of achievement in business, and while money is undoubtedly an important factor in running a professional practice, it is not the only measure of success. Prioritising personal and professional well-being, along with positive client outcomes, creates a more sustainable and fulfilling career. Be wary by being motivated only by money as this can be a fast way to alienate your clients in this service orientated profession.

Success looks different for everyone. Some may find motivation in financial growth, while others are driven by the impact they make in their clients' lives. Neither path is more valid than the other—what matters most is staying true to your own goals and values.

If external pressures ever make you question your worth, remember why you started. Focus on what truly fulfills you in your practice, and let go of comparisons that don't align with your vision. After all, this is your career, your journey, and your definition of success.

Celebrate Progress Along the Way

It's easy to become overwhelmed and demotivated by how far you have to go. Take a moment to recognise how far you've already come. Every time you learn something new—no matter how small—it's a win. And those wins add up.

When you're working toward a goal or overcoming something like Imposter Syndrome, it's easy to focus solely on what's still left to achieve. But acknowledging your progress, no matter how small it seems, can make a world of difference.

I used to brush off small wins, thinking they didn't matter unless I achieved the "final goal." But over time, I realised how much motivation and confidence I gained when I took a moment to celebrate those incremental victories. Whether it's completing a challenging task, learning something new, or simply having the courage to take a step outside your comfort zone—these moments are worth recognising.

Celebrating progress doesn't have to mean throwing a big party (though you totally can if you want!). It might look like treating yourself to a favourite meal, sharing your accomplishment with a trusted friend, or taking a moment to reflect on how far you've come. I like to write down these wins in a little book I have—it's such a great reminder on tougher days that growth is happening, even when it doesn't feel like it.

By pausing to celebrate, you're not only honouring your efforts but also reinforcing the positive habits and mindset that keep you moving forward. Don't wait for the finish line. Give yourself credit for the strides you're making right now—you've earned it.

Chapter 9: Creating Your Personalised Action Plan

The following pages are designed to guide you in writing your own personalised action plan to tackle Imposter Syndrome and move forward with confidence and purpose. Take your time with each section, reflecting deeply and answering honestly. Remember, this plan is for *you* — it's a roadmap tailored to your unique strengths, challenges, and goals.

Define Your Goals

Start by identifying what you want to achieve. Your goals could be related to overcoming specific aspects of Imposter Syndrome, personal growth, or professional development. Use the SMART criteria to make your goals Specific, Measurable, Achievable, Relevant, and Time-bound.

Example: "I want to feel confident presenting my ideas at team meetings within the next three months."

Your Goals:

_____

_____

_____

_____

_____

_____

Identify Your Strengths

Owning your strengths is a powerful step toward overcoming self-doubt. Reflect on your skills, qualities, and achievements that make you uniquely capable.

What are three strengths you bring to your personal or professional life? How have they helped you succeed in the past?

Your Strengths:

1. _____
2. _____
3. _____

_____
_____
_____
_____
_____

Pinpoint Your Triggers

Understanding what triggers your feelings of self-doubt can help you create strategies to manage them.

Think about situations where you've felt like an imposter. What were the common factors? How did you react?

Your Triggers:

1. _____
2. _____
3. _____

_____
_____
_____
_____
_____
_____
_____

Your Support System

No one overcomes challenges alone. Identify people and resources that can support your journey.

Are there colleagues, friends, or networks you can rely on for encouragement?

Your Support System:

_____

_____

_____

_____

_____

_____

_____

Create a Growth Plan

Develop habits and routines that support continuous learning and personal development.

- What gaps in your knowledge or skills would you like to address?
- What opportunities for growth can you create or pursue?

Your Plan:

Practice Gratitude and Celebrate Progress

Gratitude and recognition of your achievements can help counteract self-doubt.

- What are you grateful for in your personal and professional life?
- What small wins have you achieved recently? How will you celebrate them?

Your Gratitude List:

_____

_____

_____

_____

_____

_____

_____

Monitor and Adjust

Your action plan is a living document. Revisit it regularly to track your progress, celebrate your successes, and make adjustments as needed.

- What's working well?
- What challenges have come up?
- What new goals or strategies should you incorporate?

Your Adjustments:

_____

_____

_____

_____

_____

_____

_____

_____

Final Thoughts

You've taken the first step toward overcoming Imposter Syndrome by creating this action plan. Remember, growth takes time, and every small step counts. Keep revisiting your plan, and don't hesitate to reach out to your support system or seek additional resources when needed. You've got this!

Additional Resources

"Start where you are. The key to ongoing growth isn't to overwhelm yourself with everything—it's to start with one thing."

Books for Personal and Professional Development

***Mindset: The New Psychology of Success* by Carol S. Dweck** – A must-read on adopting a growth mindset.

***Dare to Lead* by Brené Brown** – Practical insights on courage, vulnerability, and leadership.

***Atomic Habits* by James Clear** – Powerful strategies for building habits that stick.

***The Gifts of Imperfection* by Brené Brown** – Embrace vulnerability and own your story.

***Grit: The Power of Passion and Perseverance* by Angela Duckworth** – Learn how resilience drives success.

Podcasts for Inspiration and Learning

The Tim Ferriss Show – Deep dives into habits, tools, and insights from top performers.

How to Fail with Elizabeth Day – Honest conversations about failure and resilience.

The Mindset Mentor by **Rob Dial** – Quick, actionable mindset tips.

WorkLife with Adam Grant – Explore unconventional wisdom about work and success.

Unlocking Us with Brené Brown – Real, raw conversations about being human.

Online Platforms

MassageCPE: access to online courses on various topics to help you grow as a person and in your career

Social Media Groups: Search for professional groups in your field. Join discussions and connect with like-minded professionals.

Mindfulness and Mental Wellness Tools

Headspace or Calm: Guided meditation apps to support your mental health.

Insight Timer: Free guided meditations and mindfulness practices.

Lifeline: Compassionate support for people in crisis. Call 13 11 14 (in Australia)

for 24/7 crisis support. If life is in danger, call 000.

SA Mental Health Service: For help in a mental health emergency, call the Mental Health Triage Service (in Australia) on 13 14 65 (24 hours, 7 days).

Acknowledgments

Thank you

This book was originally intended as a companion to our online course "From Self Doubt to Confidence" on www.massagecpe.com.au, but it ended up being so much more than that.

Writing this book wouldn't have been possible without the encouragement, support, and wisdom of so many wonderful people.

To my mentors—thank you for your guidance and belief in me, even when I doubted myself. You've shown me the power of mentorship firsthand and inspired me to pay it forward.

To my peers and colleagues, who have shared their stories, struggles, and triumphs—you've reminded me that none of us are alone in this journey. Your openness has been both a comfort and a catalyst for my own growth.

To my students and readers—your courage to seek self-improvement motivates me every day. Thank you for trusting me to be part of your personal and professional development.

A special thanks to my family and close friends, who are my sounding board, my cheerleaders, and my reality check when I need it most. Your unwavering support means everything to me.

Finally, to anyone who has ever struggled with self-doubt or felt like an imposter—you are the reason this book exists. I hope it serves as a reminder of your worth, your strength, and your potential.

Thank you, from the bottom of my heart, to everyone who has been part of this journey. This is as much for you as it is from me.

About the Author

Andrea is a passionate and dedicated remedial therapist and trainer and assessor. With years of hands-on experience and advanced training, she is committed to elevating the practice of massage therapy through education, advocacy, and continuous learning.

Andrea is driven by the belief that collaboration and innovation, are essential for the growth and development of the profession. Her expertise extends to writing and creating online courses, where she guides professionals in mastering techniques that enhance client care and promote self-care for therapists.

Andrea has presented at various conferences, and is actively advocating for greater recognition of massage therapists in the healthcare community. She is the author of several comprehensive courses on topics ranging from case studies to skin cancer detection, all designed to empower therapists with practical knowledge and skills.

In this book, Andrea shares her personal story about overcoming imposter syndrome to help others reach their full potential, overcome self-doubt, and foster a greater sense of confidence in their practice. Her holistic approach blends clinical expertise with a deep understanding of the personal challenges that professionals face, offering practical solutions and encouragement along the way.

When not teaching or writing, Andrea is mentoring massage therapists and contributing to the ongoing development of her field, with a firm belief that every therapist has the potential to make a meaningful difference in the lives of their clients.

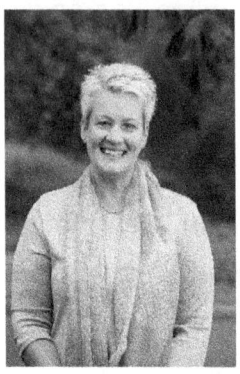

www.ingramcontent.com/pod-product-compliance
Lightning Source LLC
Chambersburg PA
CBHW070927160426
43193CB00011B/1596